Most Effective Natural Hemorrhoid Treatment

"You will not need surgery, when, you use remedies for hemorrhoids. Get relief from hemorrhoids right now."

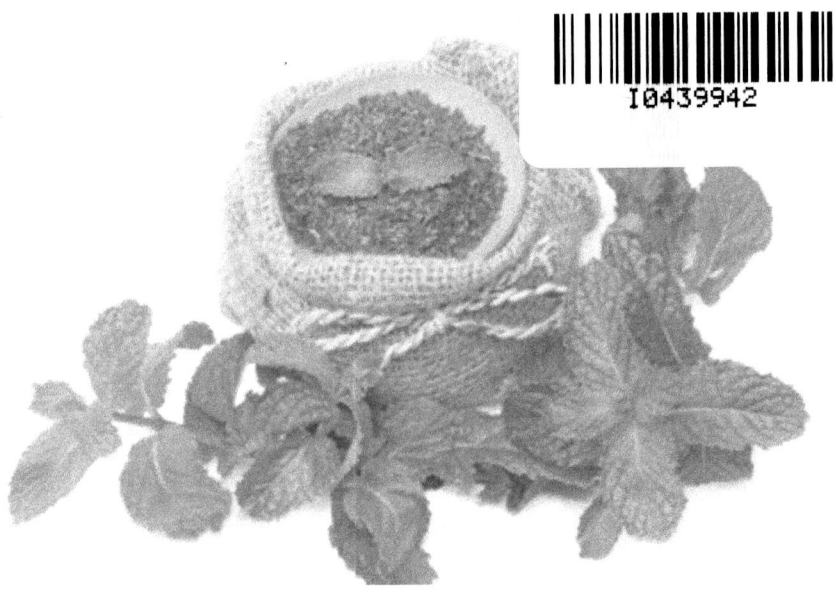

By Rudy S Silva, Natural Nutritionist

Most Effective Natural Hemorrhoid Treatment © 2011
updated 2014 by Rudy S Silva

ISBN-13: 978-1481101998
ISBN-10: 1481101994

Disclaimer and Terms of Use: The Author and Publisher has strived to be as accurate and complete as possible in the creation of this book, although he does not warrant or represent at any time that the contents within are accurate due to the rapidly changing nature of the Internet. While all attempts have been made to verify information provided in this publication, the Author and Publisher assume no responsibility for errors, omissions, or contrary interpretation of the subject matter herein. Any perceived slights of specific persons, peoples, or organizations are unintentional. In practical advice books, like anything else in life, there are no guarantees of income made. This book is not intended for use as a source of legal, business, accounting, or medical. All readers are advised to seek services of competent professionals in legal, business, accounting, and medical field.

First Printing in the United States of America

Table of Contents

1: What You Need To Know About Hemorrhoids

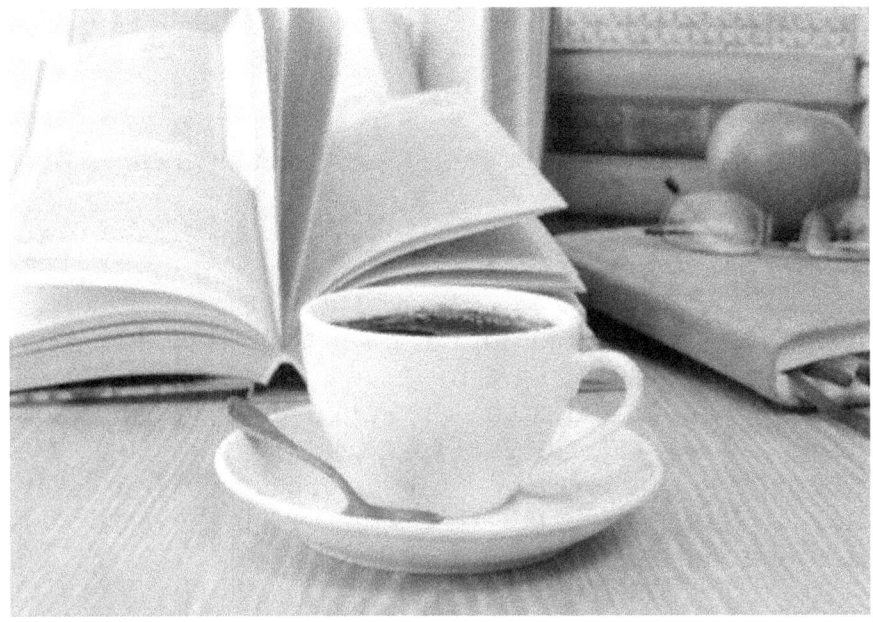

There are many unpleasant symptoms and diseases associated with constipation. Hemorrhoids are one such symptom, and many doctors or practitioners say, "It's not a serious condition." As a natural nutritional consultant, I say, "Hemorrhoids is a condition you need to reduce or better yet eliminate." And, this can be done with natural methods.

To keep yourself healthy and prevent illness and disease to take hold, you need to listen to all symptoms or pain your body develops. Sometimes just acknowledging a simple symptom is enough for it and the cause to disappear. Hemorrhoids, whether simple or severe, are your body's ways of telling you there is something wrong somewhere, and "I hope you take care of it before it gets worse"

Taking care of hemorrhoids or its symptoms is just part of what you want to do. You want to concentrate part of your effort on getting to the cause. If you eliminate the cause of hemorrhoids, it will be easier to get rid of them.

The first signs of hemorrhoids are when you need to take action. Don't wait until your hemorrhoids get large, give you pain, start bleeding, or protrude.

The first question you should ask about hemorrhoids is what caused them.

What causes hemorrhoids?

It is always the cause of an illness that you should be after. Doctors don't usually have the time to determine what the cause is, so they will treat the symptom or get rid of it for you. It's up to you to take charge of your health. I know you are this type of person; otherwise, you would not be reading this book. Hemorrhoids are caused by excess pressure in the rectal veins and veins in the surrounding area.

There are many causes of hemorrhoids of which constipation is a major cause. Work on eliminating your hemorrhoid symptoms, using the natural remedies listed in this book. At the same time, work on getting rid of constipation, so that you can be free of hemorrhoids and the other diseases that could follow.

In their book, Natural Prescriptions, 1994, Robert M. Giller, M.D. and Kathy Matthews, gives you their opinion of drugstore medications,

"If you are suffering from hemorrhoids right now, you want immediate relief. What about all those over-the-counter remedies? Just last year the FDA clamped down on the manufacturers of these products, and some of them are being removed from the market because they've never been proven to be effective. Other must limit their claims. Those that claim to shrink tissues must carry a warning because people with diabetes or heart disease, for example, shouldn't use them. In the final analysis, while you may get some temporary relief from these products, you could do as well by applying zinc oxide, petroleum jelly, or witch hazel, which are just as effective and far cheaper."

Many different natural remedies for reducing, relieving, and eliminating hemorrhoids are listed here. Since everyone is different in their chemical make-up and nutritional requirements, one remedy will not work for everyone. Each of you has to find out what remedy works best for you. Use the remedy that feels right for you, the remedy where you have the ingredients, or the one based on the severity of your hemorrhoids.

What are hemorrhoids?

Constipation, Hemorrhoids or Piles, and inactivity go hand in hand. If you have been constipated for quite a while, chances are you have hemorrhoids. If you are inactive because you just like sitting around or are confined to a bed or chair, then you will have constipation and hemorrhoids.

The diet and preventative measures to take for hemorrhoids are the same for constipation. Eliminating constipation is the first step in curing your hemorrhoids. The next step is using natural remedies to eliminate your hemorrhoids. The third step is to increase your activity through walking, exercise, or other moving activities.

These three steps can be done at the same time especially if you have hemorrhoids that are itchy or painful and are in need of attention.

Constipation

Constipation occurs when the fecal matter remains in your colon 25 hours or more. You should be having at least one and two bowel movements per day and two is better, especially if you are eating three meals a day. If you are not then, you are constipated to the point where you may need to puff, push, or strain to have a bowel movement.

Bowel movements must occur naturally. When your colon is working well, and you are eating good food, then you will have the urge to have 1-2-3 bowel movements per day. If you do not have 2-3 bowel movements per day, don't worry and don't force yourself to have them. Just start changing your diet, as I have outlined in the following chapters and as time passes you will have more natural bowel movements during the day. One to two bowel movements per day is natural and three if you eat a lot during the day.

Enlarged Veins

Hemorrhoids, in the rectum, occur when the veins are not returning enough blood back to the heart. When this happens, the vein walls do not receive enough oxygen and release a substance into the blood that causes them swell and become inflamed. This swelling causes the vein to become weakened and more likely to break when they are rubbed, like during a bowel movement.

If your stools are hard, you have a higher chance of breaking a swelling vein. For this reason getting your stools softer is one step in clearing your hemorrhoids. You can do this by eating a healthy diet and using remedies that are directed at relieving constipation.

Hemorrhoids are on the inside just above the muscle that

closes the anus and goes into to the rectum. They are near the surface of the rectum mucus membrane on the outside. They occur on the skin that surrounds the anus and protrude or hangs outward.

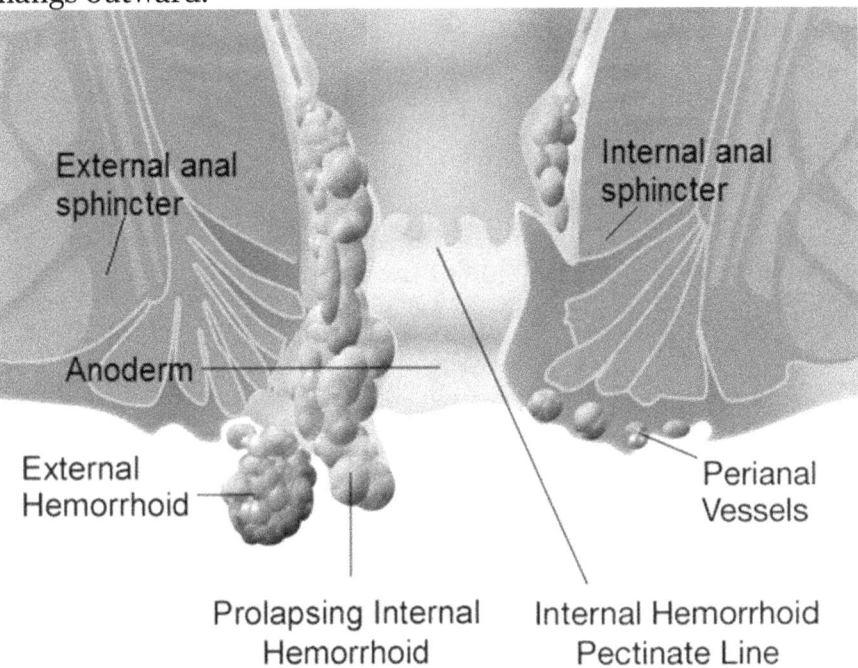

External anal sphincter

Internal anal sphincter

Anoderm

External Hemorrhoid

Perianal Vessels

Prolapsing Internal Hemorrhoid

Internal Hemorrhoid Pectinate Line

On the outside, they are called a prolapsed hemorrhoid, when they occur inside on the rectum and come through the anus and hang outward. In a way, hemorrhoids can be considered varicose veins of the rectum. Just like varicose veins in the legs, the rectum veins become enlarged and come to the skin surface and bulge out.

Hemorrhoids occur when you are constipated for long periods, sit for many hours, lift heavy items, or are pregnant. If you're constipated, you're probably having a difficult time having a bowel movement. And when you do, your stools are usually small, hard, or dry. If you have to push and strain or sit on the toilet for 10-15 minutes, then expect to have hemorrhoids at some point. Two to three minutes is all you normally need to have a natural bowel movement.

Over 85% of the population has hemorrhoids. Hemorrhoids are a sign that fecal matter is not passing through your colon like it should. Simple hemorrhoids are not dangerous to your health, but hemorrhoids that have been building for a while will cause you some discomfort, such as,

- Mucus discharge
- Bleeding showing up in your stools or dripping into the toilet water
- Itching on the outside of the rectum
- Pain in the rectum area and during a bowel movement
- Pain in the rectum area, when you sit the soft bulging area in the rectum or anus that give you a sensation that something is there

Health Alert: See your doctor, if your hemorrhoids are painful, have excess bleeding, or stools have change in color from medium brown to dark brown or black.

Hemorrhoids typically don't itch. If they itch only at night, you may have pinworms.

In her book, Digestive Wellness, 1996, Elizabeth Lipski, M.S.,C.C.N, tells you how to check for pinworms,

"Place a piece of tape around your finger, sticky side out. Put the tape on your anus, pull it off and check for worms, which look like moving white threads. If you are checking one of your children, you can use the tape method or just look. Another cause of rectal itching is called pruritus ani which can be caused by food sensitivities, contact with irritating substance (laundry detergent or toilet paper), fungi, bacterial infection, parasites, antibiotics, poor hygiene or tight clothing."

How Hemorrhoids are Formed

Veins move blood back to the heart, and arteries move blood to various parts of the body from the heart. So, veins that surround the rectum and anus take away cellular waste from this area to the liver to be detoxified.

When you have a bowel movement, the veins in the rectum and anus expand and return to normal when you finish. When you have constipation and you push and strain to have a bowel movement, the veins along the rectum and anus have increased pressure.

Over a period of time, these veins become weaken, lose their tone and can become permanently swollen and large. This swelling is the source of itching and pain, when the veins touch nearby nerves. If the veins become large enough they can block the passage of fecal matter.

What do Hemorrhoids Cause in Your Body?

Hemorrhoids do not cause any specific disease or illness in the short term. However, if you do not treat them, they can become large, block fecal matter, bleed and be a source of additional inflammation. If not treated, in severe cases, they can become a source of bacterial infection with severe pain and discomfort. Then, they can become the place where serious disease can form.

Hemorrhoids occur in stages:

Hemorrhoids are slightly enlarged veins either in the rectum or on the anus. They do not hang down and generally do not bleed. They are in the starting stages of expanding veins and can be seen and felt.

Hemorrhoids are not prolapsed (coming out of the rectum and hanging) but when you strain to have a bowel movement, they swell and decrease when you finish your bowel movement. Hemorrhoids are excessive prolapsed with straining. They push out of the rectum and hang out. They can be pushed back into the rectum. They bleed when you have a bowel movement. Large hemorrhoids protrude out of the rectum all the time and bleed all the time.

The more severe your hemorrhoids are the more likely they will bleed.

Many years ago, I noticed blood in the toilet water after having a bowel movement. The cause was bleeding from hemorrhoids, but my doctor didn't notice this right away. The result was he had me go through a barium enema to see if I had internal bleeding. This process is not painful but was definitely uncomfortable.

How do you get them?

Constipation is the main cause of hemorrhoids. But, constipation is not the only way that you can get hemorrhoids. Here are some additional ways:

- Alcoholism
- Being pregnant
- Doing daily heavy lifting and holding your breath while you do it
- Eating foods that are bad for your health and cause constipation
- General body weakness
- Having a predisposition to constipation
- Inheriting a weakness in the colon and rectum area
- Having a weak liver

- Irregular eating patterns
- Lack of protein leading to weak tissues and slow healing of wounds
- Not eating foods that keep you constipation free
- Not getting the right vitamins and minerals in your food
- Being overweight
- Poor muscle tone in the anal area from lack of exercise
- Pressure on rectum veins from cysts or tumor in the colon
- Sexual excess
- Sitting in a chair at home, at work, in a car, or in a truck for long periods
- Using laxatives to the point where your colon no longer works right, and you end up with constipation.

2: Medical Treatment For Hemorrhoids

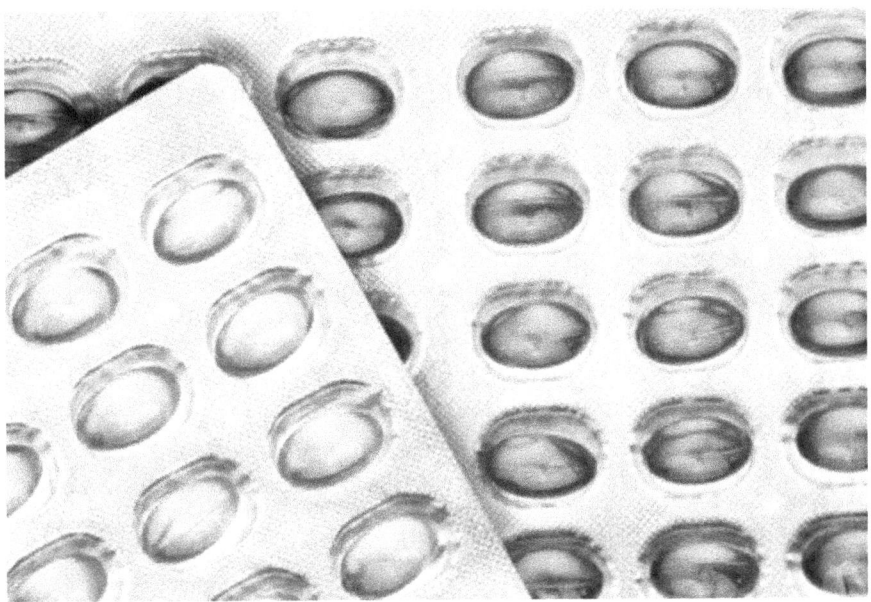

Drugstore hemorrhoid medications

There are many drug stores and alternative Internet products for treating hemorrhoids. Most of the products are not made to cure or eliminate hemorrhoids but to give you temporary relief of itching, pain, swelling or bleeding. I don't recommend using any type of product that is not natural.

If the product contains petrochemicals, additives, coloring, dyes, or other chemicals, which enhance its appearance and feel, I would not use them. Most, if not all, of these chemicals will be absorbed into your body where your organs of elimination will have to deal with eliminating them.

All products, whether drugs, drugstore medications, or natural formulations use chemicals, substances, oils, and herbs that have these properties,

- Anesthetics – suppresses pain and gives relief...any name with the suffix "caine" like tetracaine.
- Analgesics – suppresses and gives pain relief – some of them are Anacin, Tylenol with Codeine, OxyContin,
- Vasoconstrictors – helps to narrow or constrict hemorrhoidal veins...any name with the suffix "rine" like phenylephrine
- Lubricants – provide lubrication in the colon to relieve constipation – mineral oil, flax seed oil, castor oil, olive oil.
- Astringents – helps to tighten the tissue which has been pushed out by hemorrhoids – zinc oxide, witch hazel, and calamine.
- Keratolytics – helps to remove excess hemorrhoidal tissue.

Many of the drugstore medications have anesthetics. They can aggravate and irritate the hemorrhoids you're trying to eliminate. If you are using one of these drugstore medications, consider using a more natural remedy.

In 1975 Carl I. Flath, wrote a book called The Miracle Nutrient – How Dietary Fiber Can Save Your Life. In his book, he talks about the effectiveness of drugstore suppositories, "Suppositories quickly work their way up in the rectum beyond the location of the most internal hemorrhoids, and so are of limited value in reducing local pain. As antiseptics, they are essentially worthless, since the surface areas, they are supposed to protect are under constant exposure to new bacteria.... Anesthetic agents do offer temporary relief from local irritations and pain... Neither the suppositories nor the ointments, however, do anything whatever to correct the basic cause of hemorrhoids—constipation."

Hemorrhoid Surgery

For severe hemorrhoids, surgery may be the only way to get rid of them. However, there are many antidotal stories of people who have used some of the remedies listed here and avoided surgery.

You have to decide how you want to clear your hemorrhoids. The following chapters give you a choice of what to do.

3: How To Use Herbs For Hemorrhoids

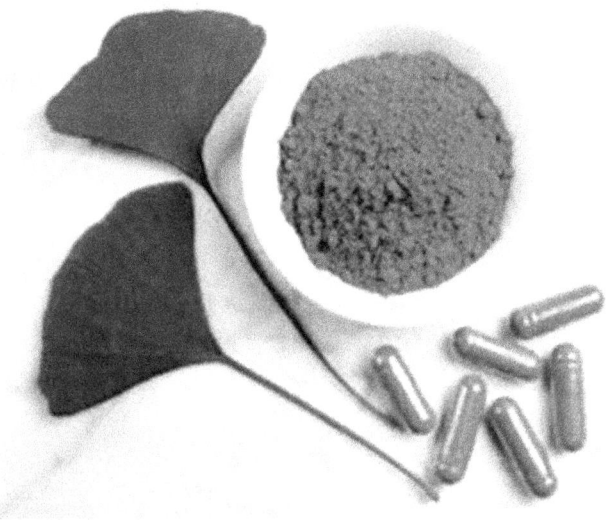

To get rid of hemorrhoids, first look at the ways listed to get your bowels moving easier and more frequently, so they produce softer stools. Any straining and puffing you do to push hard or soft stools out, during a bowel movement will aggravate your hemorrhoids and can lead to bleeding and pain.

When completing a bowel movement, make sure you are using the softest tissue available, so that when you clean yourself, you do not scrape or aggravate your hemorrhoids. You can also use pre- moisten tissue. Just make sure that the tissue you use is not colored or scented because these chemical additives can aggravate your hemorrhoids. You may have to take a shower a couple of times a day to keep your anus area clean.

Here is a list of the natural remedies that you can use to aid in eliminating your hemorrhoids.

Aloe Vera

Aloe Vera gel is an astringent that helps to heal open wounds. It is useful in hemorrhoids by applying the gel directly onto your anus and slightly into your rectum. The best type of gel for this is directly from the aloe plant. If you don't have one, then 100% organic whole leaf aloe gel is second best. You can get this aloe at a health food or nutrition store. In some cases, the gel may be 99% pure with another herb added and this is ok.

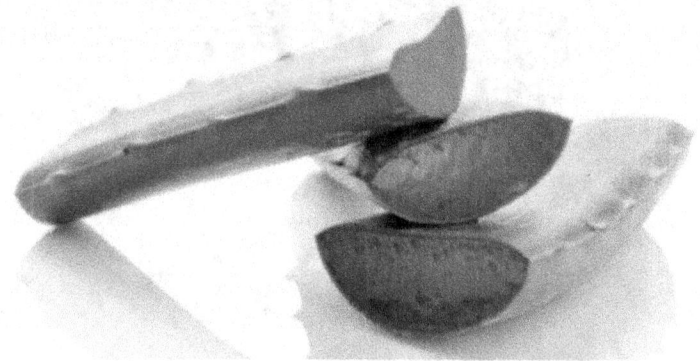

If you have a fresh plant, cut and wash a leaf thoroughly with distilled water. Remove the sharp sticker on both sides. Then, peel it on one side, bend it with the peeled side outward, and slip it into your anus. This will provide you with pain relief and reduce your hemorrhoid bleeding. Just trim down the leaf so it slides into your anus easily.

Aloe Vera juice that you drink is also good for hemorrhoids. It helps to soften your stools and to activate peristaltic action. If you like aloe juice, then drink around 1/2 a cup of Aloe Vera juice three times a day.

You can add 1/4 or 1/3 part aloe juice to a cup of apple juice to make the taste easier to handle.

To make this aloe-apple juice more effective, add 10 drops of barberry extract.
Barberry is an astringent for blood vessel congestion along the colon and rectum. It will improve blood circulation; it stimulates the immune system to resist disease, and will tone body tissues. It also is capable of stopping bleeding hemorrhoids.

You can also use aloe vera capsules, which will help with your digestion and constipation. Go here for the capsules.

Botanic Choice Aloe Vera

Or here, http://tinyurl.com/ll3j26q

Bilberry

Bilberry's active ingredients are flavonoids. Bilberry contains chemical called "anthocyanosides." This fruit like herb has been used in Europe for a long time. In clinical studies, it has shown to be effective in treating weak capillaries by strengthening their walls.

Buy the 25% standardized formula and take 100 mg three times a day of bilberry.

Vitacost Bilberry Extract – Standardized

Or, http://tinyurl.com/kjyvc69

Butcher's Broom

Butcher's broom, an evergreen bush, has a history of being used for varicose veins and hemorrhoids. As an extract, it contains "ruscogenins", which can narrow blood vessels and decrease their inflammation and swelling. It strengthens and tones veins and capillary walls.

Take 100 mg of butcher's broom three times a day. Use the type has 9-11% ruscogenins.

Solgar FP Butcher's Broom Vegetable Capsules or

http://tinyurl.com/kxzqkxe

Collinsonia Root Powder Or Extract

Collinsonia is a vegetable, known as "Stone Root" because of it hardness. It comes in powder and liquid. Stone Root is found in Canada and in Florida. It has been found quite helpful in hemorrhoids. Used over time this herb strengthens the veins.

Collinsonia is an astringent and antispasmodic that gives relief and prevents hemorrhoids. It improves blood circulation in capillaries, and this makes the membranes in the rectum more relaxed and stable. In addition, it will strengthen weak tissue, especially in the capillaries and veins.

Linda Clark in her book called, Linda Clark's Handbook of natural remedies for common ailments, 1976, says this about Collinsonia root.

"I have heard people rave enthusiastically about the results of this remedy, which works quickly."

Collinsonia benefits come from, supporting blood vessel contractions and flow reducing irritation and inflammation of veins, providing a tonic effect on weaken veins, capillaries, and tissue.

Here's how to use it.

If you use the extract, take 6-12 drops in juice or water, and swish in your mouth for a few seconds. Do this 3 times a day. It the extract in a dark place and keep away from children. If you are pregnant or a nursing woman do not use Collinsonia.

If you buy Collinsonia powder in capsules, you just take 3 capsules three times every day with a large glass of water. Also, use arrowroot for symptom relief while you are using the Collinsonia capsules by dabbing some arrowroot powder on the area a few times daily.

Here is a website where you can get Collinsonia powder capsules,

Collinsonia or **http://tinyurl.com/nrl7k8o**

Comfrey powder

Comfrey powder or (**http://tinyurl.com/muchslx**) comes from an herbal root that has plenty of allantoin. This herb is a powerful acting herb that is anti- inflammatory and stimulates the formation of new skin. It can also cause hemorrhoids that are outside of the anus to shrink and pull back.

Here's how to use it.

Buy the powder and not the liquid. Make a paste by mixing it with olive, fish, or flaxseed oil. Apply the paste directly onto your anus and surrounding area. You can apply it at night, and your morning shower will remove it. Fresh comfrey leaves or roots are the best to use. However, you can get precut and dried comfrey from a health-food store. If you use the dried leaves, you can put them into a coffee grinder to create a powder. Use this powder to create a paste with oils.

Gotu Kola

Gotu Kola is an India herb that is a hemorrhoidal remedy. Use an extract that has 70% triterpenic acid since this is the active ingredient.

Gotu kola extract reduces pain, swelling, fatigue, and

sensation of heaviness from hemorrhoids.

Get the extract here,

Botanic Choice Liquid Extract, Gotu Kola or,
http://tinyurl.com/kb4d3b4

Horse Chestnut

Horse chestnut comes from the bark of a tree and has been found useful in treating hemorrhoids. It contains the chemicals "aesculin" and "aescin" that strengthen your blood vessels and which help to reduce hemorrhoids. It also helps to reduce inflamed areas.

Nature's Way Horse chestnut Standardized Extract or
http://tinyurl.com/mk3pa3f

Here's how to use it.

You can make a tea and apply it directly to your hemorrhoids. However, do not drink the tea since it contains tannin, which tighten mucus and tissue and would cause constipation.

Use it in powder form and mix it with olive oil or other oils to produce a paste and apply it to your anus area.

Also, you can open the capsules for the powder to make the paste. You can also take the capsules as directed on the bottle, one capsule twice a day.

Plantain Herb

Plantain also has plenty of allantoin just like comfrey root powder.

Here's how to use it.

Use it just like comfrey powder by mixing it with oil and applying it directly to your anus.

You can also combine equal parts of the plantain and comfrey powder. If you only have plantain leaves, put them in a coffee grinder to create a powder. Now you can make a mixture with oil and both herbs.

Plantain Powder Organic or http://tinyurl.com/m5e8j3r

Prickly Ash Bark

Prickly ash bark has been successfully used to cure or eliminate hemorrhoids. It is an astringent, antiseptic, tonic, and stimulant of blood and lymphatic system.

Health Alert: If pregnant, don't use prickly ash bark since it simulates peristaltic action.

Here's where you can get it.

Prickly Ash Bark Product Website

Witch Hazel

Witch hazel comes in liquid or gel and gives a "cool relief" feeling and provides astringent action. You can apply witch hazel directly to your anus. You can also prepare a pad moistened with witch hazel and place it on your bottom and leave it over night or during the day.

Witch hazel is used in many drugstore preparations. It is much cheaper to use pure witch hazel and create your own moisten pads. Let's go onto the next chapter.

Using Liquid Herbal Extracts

In his book called Therapeutic Herb Manual, 2004, Ed Smith answers the question,

"How is the best way to take liquid herbal extracts?

Generally I prefer to mix the prescribed number of extract drops into 2 to 4 ounces of water. You can also add the drops to warm tea (not hot) or juice. Certain herbs, because of their stronger action, require more water and these have been so noted under 'dose' in this manual. For optimal results sip the mixed drops so you can savor the extract's flavor and aroma, although you may not always like the taste."

4: Using Herbal Combinations For Hemorrhoids

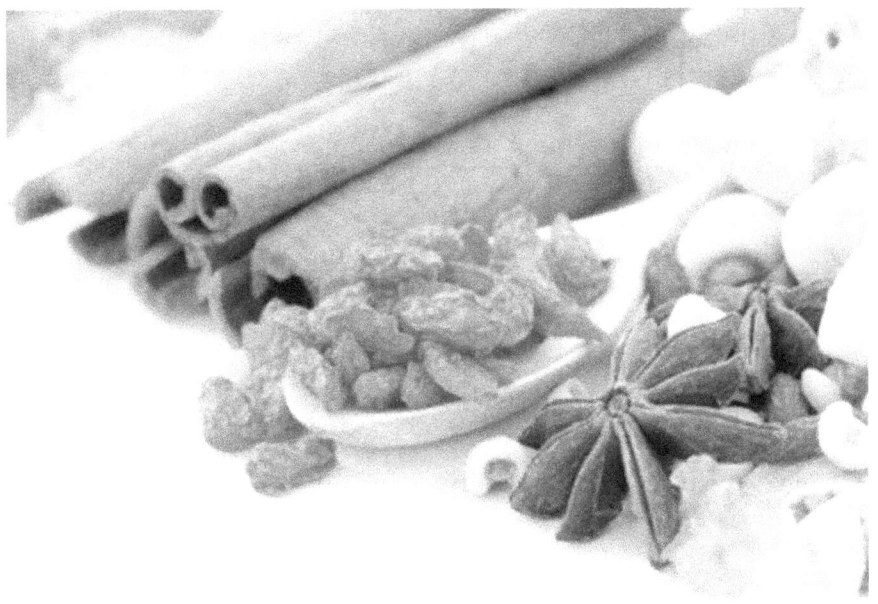

Asian Herbs

I have found Chinese's herb formulation quite effective. It is now easy to find these herbs, since there are Chinese's herb stores in most cities. If not, it is easy to go to the Internet and find what you need.

These herbs normally come in pill form; however, you can also get store owners to mix you a formulation of dried herbs by simply telling them what ailment you are trying to treat. Some Chinese herbal stores have an acupuncturist that can diagnose your problem and prescribe for an herbal combination.

These Chinese hemorrhoid herbs contain chemicals that are anti- inflammatory, antiseptic, increase blood circulation, and lift Chi. Chi is the life force that powers all body and mind functions. When checking these Chinese formulations just make sure the manufacturers note that they are low in heavy metals.

FARGELIN – is a Chinese herbal formulation that is used for painful hemorrhoids with swelling and redness. It also cools the blood and invigorates it.

This formulation has been used for centuries with great results in China and Russia. It has been used eliminate hemorrhoids gently, quickly and safely.

Use three tablets per day.

Go to this site, **http://tinyurl.com/nnt8s9a** to see how this Chinese formulation's ingredients and its price.

HUA ZHI LING WAN (hemorrhoid pills) this product is the same as Fargelin.

HUAI JIAO WAN – shrinks, reduces pain, and stops **bleeding of hemorrhoids**

JING WAN HUNG – relieves pain burning and itching of hemorrhoids. or

http://www.modernherbshop.com/Ching_Wan_Hun g_Burn_Ointment_p/burnointment.htm Collinsonia – Horse Chestnut Compound

Here is a liquid extract that contains many of the herbs that are good for stabilizing and improving the tone of the veins around the rectum and anus. It contains the following herbs:

• Collinsonia

- Horse Chestnut seed
- Butcher's Broom
- Rosemary flowering branches
- Prickly as bark

Here's how to use it,

As a preventative, use 20-30 drops in water one to two times per day.

For use in a good case of hemorrhoids, use 30-40 drops in water three times per day.

For a severe case of hemorrhoids, use 40-50 drops in water, three to five times per day.

Do not exceed 150 drops within one day. When using herbs, it is best to use the cycle of,

Use 6 days per week, 6weeks, and rest for one week, and then continue the cycle again. Here's where to get it,

Collinsonia – **Horse Chestnut Compound** or
http://tinyurl.com/mkzdenk

Health alert: when using Horse Chestnut in any herbal mixture, consult your health practitioner before using it, if you're pregnant or nursing, or have of liver or kidney diseases.

Pilex Tablets and Ointment

Pilex is an India formulation that contains many herbs. It is used for only seven days and has been found to give relief from hemorrhoids for up to six months.

To get complete information on this product and dose, go to, You can check out this site for the ingredients of both pilex tablets and ointment or http://tinyurl.com/ogaxhwv .

Swedish Bitters

Here is a hemorrhoid herbal extract formulation called Swedish bitter.

Aloe

Myrrh

Saffron

Senna leaves

Camphor

Rhubarb roots

Manna

Theriac venezian

Carline Thistle roots

Angelica roots

Zedoary roots

This formulation relieves hemorrhoidal pain, burning, and itching. Soak a cotton ball in **Swedish bitters** and apply it directly your hemorrhoids.

You can find it at this website.

http://tinyurl.com/mhobekm

Herbs for Hemorrhoids

Here is a list of herbs to look for in the ointments or hemorrhoid products you buy.

- Slippery elm – has a soothing effect on body areas that

are inflamed, swelling, and ulcerous. It has adhesive glue like property that is good for relieving hemorrhoids.

- Witch hazel – contains tannic acid with helps to produce its astringent property. It helps to constrict or pull together hemorrhoids that are bulging.
- Mullein – soothes irritated mucus surfaces or open skin areas. It reduces pain and swelling.
- Wild alum root – also known as cranes bill root. It is a strong astringent. It works to reduce hemorrhoidal irritation and provides veins with chemicals that give it tone and strength.
- Goldenseal root – constrict blood vessels, which allow hemorrhoids to shrink and to give them time to heal.

5: How To Shrink Hemorrhoids With Ointments

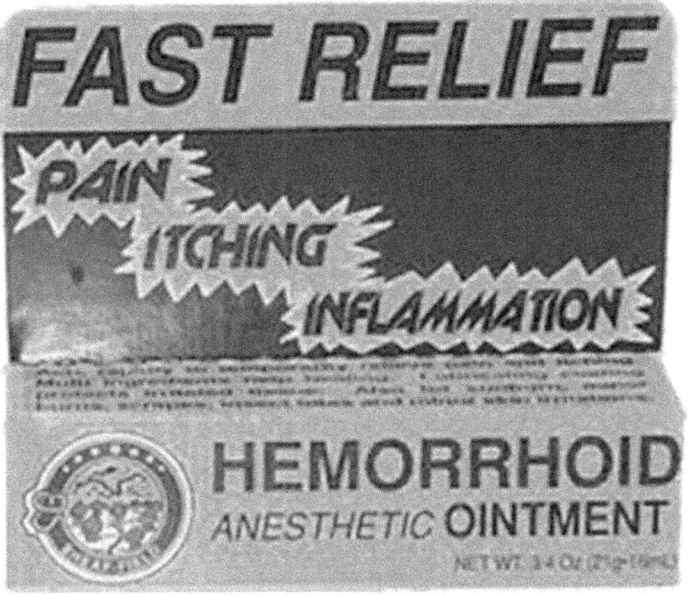

Comfrey Herbal Salve

Here an herbal combination that contains herbs that promote the healing of skin wounds and blood vessel, is antiseptic, anti-inflammatory, analgesic, soothing, and anti-itching, **comfrey root ointment** or **http://tinyurl.com/kc26pmb**

Here's how to use it,

Clean the area where you want to apply the salve. Apply the salve to the anus or slightly into the rectum by rubbing to soften the salve. This application can be done at night so that you get a good dose of this salve.

Use six days on and six weeks on with one-week rest.

When using any kind of salve and herbal extracts, keep them in the refrigerator. This keeps them fresh and gives your hemorrhoid a "cool relief" Feeling.

Here is another **comfrey ointment** from Cloverleaf Farms, **http://www.cloverleaffarmherbsandgifts.com/produ ct/MGONcoo2.html**

Veri-Gone salve

Here's a salve that was made for varicose veins and has been used for general cases of hemorrhoids.
Witch Hazel

Echinacea Extract

Calendula Extract

Chamomile essential oil

Alcohol

Distilled water

Here's where you can find this salve. This site has a variety of salve formulation.

Veri-Gone Website

Ghee – Turmeric Salve
Here's a Ghee mixture that is listed in, New Choices in Natural Healing, 1995, by Prevention Magazine Health Books.

Combine 1 teaspoon of ghee with 1/2 teaspoon of turmeric powder. Apply some of this mixture onto your hemorrhoids just before you go to bed.

Here's how to use it,
Apply it for 3 nights in a row

Stop for two nights
Resume for three nights

Continue this cycle until your hemorrhoids are gone.

Wear old clothes when you use this combination since the turmeric will stain your clothes. The discoloration on your skin will clear after two-three weeks or sooner.

Zinc Oxide Ointment

Zinc Oxide is readily available in a drugstore or throughout the Internet. It is useful in reducing hemorrhoids symptoms since it is astringent, antiseptic, and antibacterial.

Zinc oxide will keep the area dry from moisture and will help to reduce itching and chafing. Use it as often as you like and, of course, when you go to bed.

Calendula Ointment

Calendula flower has been extensive used in China to heal hemorrhoids. It has a soothing effect and reduces inflammation. Its other characteristics are,

- Antibacterial

- Analgesic

- Antiseptic

- Astringent

- hemostatic (stops bleeding)

- styptic (contracts blood vessels)

- Tissue Forming

Apply the ointment directly on your hemorrhoids. Use it daily and as often as you like. Here's where to get it,
Calendula Ointment or http://tinyurl.com/megl45g

Shepherd's Purse

Shepherd's purse is used to stop bleeding. When taken as a tea, it will help stop internal bleeding whatever it comes in contact with. This is not an ointment. It's a tea that you use directly on your hemorrhoids.

Here's how to make the tea,

Take 3 tablespoons of shepherd's purse herb and put it into a glass container with 2 cups of distilled water. Bring this mixture to boil, and then bring the mixture to where it is just simmering. Allow some of the water to evaporate for about 10 minutes. Now strain the solution and allow it to cool.

Drink ¼ of a cup of this tea or more. Then moisten gauze with this tea and press it against your anus for about 10 minutes, or until you get the results, you want.

6: Other Remedies For Quick Hemorrhoid Relief

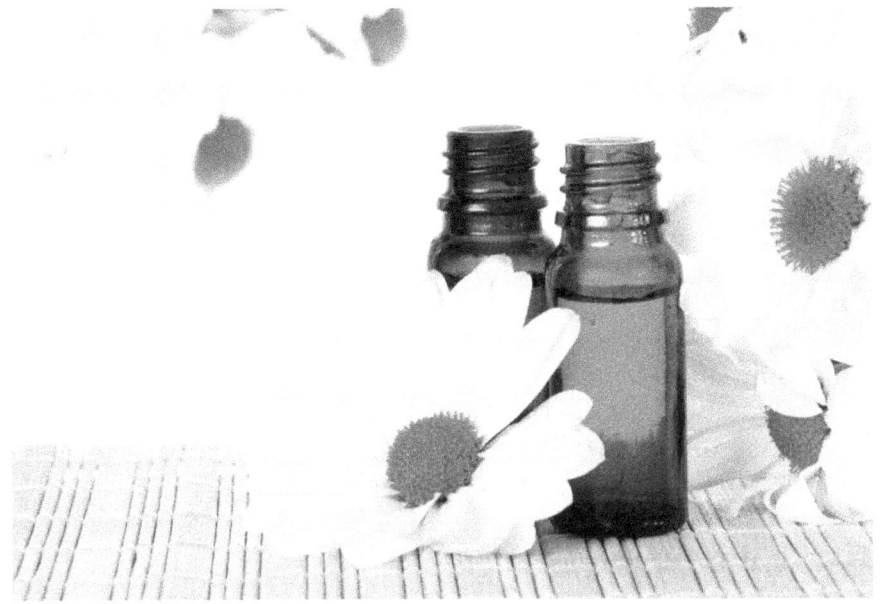

Bromelain

Bromelain is a digestive enzyme that is found in pineapple. It's capable of reducing inflammation and swelling, and for this reason, it has been used to treat hemorrhoids.

Bromelian also activates a chemical that promotes the breakdown of fibrin. Fibrin is a chemical that repairs open wounds, internal wounds and weak tissue by creating fibrin deposits. By over doing its job, fibrin causes sickness, disease, and inflammation and needs to be dissolved by systemic enzymes – enzymes that exist in the blood and though out the body. But, systemic enzymes are also available in capsules.

Take 500-750 mg of bromelain a day. You can also add fresh pineapple to your diet, since it is high in fiber and other nutrients.

Calendula Flower Bath

Here's how to prepare this flower bath. In a tub of water, add 6-8 calendula flowers and 3 tablespoons of Epsom salts. Soak yourself in this water for about 15-20 minutes.

You can buy calendula-dried flowers wherever they sell dried herbs.

Calendula promotes healing of wounds and tissue. It stops bleeding, pain, and skin irritations. It is also an astringent.

Chlorophyll

Chlorophyll is a wonder liquid, since detoxifies your body and builds your blood. Using chlorophyll regularly will help you keep your blood strong and bring more oxygen to your cells and those areas that are in need of regenerating.

Here's how to use it,

Daily, mix 2-3 tablespoon of liquid chlorophyll with the juice of one lemon in 8 oz of distilled water. Take it first thing in the morning.

Cranberry Poultice

For relief of hemorrhoids within an hour, here what you can do,

- Blend 3-4 tablespoons of raw cranberries.
- Wrap a tablespoon of this blend or so in some cheesecloth.
- Push it up against your anus and keep it there with some tight underwear.
- After an hour or so replace it with a new batch of berries and cloth.
- Apply these berries twice and do it the next day if necessary.

Digestive and Systemic Enzymes

Digestive enzymes are used to help you digest your food and improve your assimilation. Systemic enzymes are found deep into your body. They are in your tissues, organs, and cells where they help in all types of chemical reactions.

Both these enzymes are available in capsules to supplement your diet.

Digestive enzymes help to reduce the stress you get in the rectum, when your food is not properly digested. Undigested food reaching the colon eventually leads to constipation.

Take a good digestive enzyme that you can get at a health food store. Take 2 capsules with each meal.

Systemic enzymes help reduce swelling, inflammation, improve circulation, and speed the healing of tissue. One important fact about systemic enzymes is they eliminate fibrin, which is at the center of most inflammatory conditions and illness.

Take systemic enzymes between meals. This allows them to reach the small intestine and gets absorbed into the blood stream where they can do their work. If you take them with meals, they will get used up in the stomach, digesting food.

Some systemic enzymes are an enteric enzyme, which means they are coated so they will not dissolve in the stomach. This allows them to move into the small intestine, where they will be absorbed into your blood stream.

Here are the systemic enzymes you should use, Vitalzym. It contains serrapeptase, a powerful systemic enzyme.
It can be purchased at:

Vitalzym Capsules or go to http://tinyurl.com/lztutkf

Essential Oil for hemorrhoids

Certain essential oils can be used for hemorrhoids by mixing them with almond oil. This mixture can then be used in the anus area.

Here are the oils to use.

- Almond – is a carrier oil for the other oils, help to reduce pain, promotes clean skin

- Cypress - is antiseptic, astringent, soothing, reduces pain

- Juniper – is antiseptic, reduces pain

- Lavender – repairs wounds, reduces swelling, antiseptic

- Lemon – bactericide, antiseptic, repels parasites, stringent, reduces inflammation

- Rosemary – antiseptic, reduces pain, stimulates blood flow

Use essential oils only on top of the skin and do not use them internally since these oils can be toxic. Use Almond oil as carrier oil with any of the oils you use.

A combination that you can make is:
- One once of almond oil

- Three drops of cypress oil

- Three drops of rosemary oil

- Three drops of lavender oil

Place these oils in a dark-brown dropper one-ounce bottle. You can mix other combinations. You may have to experiment to see what works for you. This is part of taking control of your health.

Geranium-Lavender Essential Oil Mixture

Combine 2-3 drops of lavender to one and two drop of geranium oil with one ounce of almond oil. Place this combination in a dark-brown bottle with a dropper top. After shaking this combination, use a few drops on your fingers and apply it directly on the skin surrounding your anus.

Garlic and Onions

Garlic and onions can be used as a suppository. Using them will help to strengthen the veins, kill bacteria in the area, and reduce inflammation.

Peel a small garlic or onion. Reduce the size of the onion to a garlic clove size. Just before bed you can push either garlic or onion just lightly into your rectum, but not too far in. Your regular bowel movement will remove them in the morning.

Health Alert: Do not use this method, if your hemorrhoids have been bleeding or are bleeding. Wait for this area to heal.

Liquid Lecithin

Apply liquid lecithin to the hemorrhoids one to two times a day. Do this for 2-3 days. Continue its use until you get the relief you want from your hemorrhoids.

Ice Pack

To get quick relief from hemorrhoidal pain and swelling, prepare an ice pack as follows:

Make your own ice pack by putting ice cubes or crushed ice into a plastic bag. Wrap the plastic bag with a thin piece of cloth. Place the ice pack into the hemorrhoid area.

You can also use the slim commercial ice gels pack. Cover it with a thin piece of cloth and place it into the hemorrhoid area. Apply the ice pack for 15-20 minutes, then rest for 10-15 minutes. Continue applying the ice pack for another 15-20 minutes. Do this for 2-3 hours. Then, take a rest for 2-3 hours, then start again.

Health Tip: Don't put ice or ice gel pack directly on your skin without wrapping it with a cloth.

Lemon Juice and Papaya Skins

Use lemon juice or papaya skins against your anus to reduce or eliminate itching. You can make lemon drink that can help strengthen capillaries and blood vessel walls. Here's how to do it,

Use an organic lemon since you will be using the outer peel. Slice the lemon into 4 parts – don't peel the lemon. Use the whole lemon.

Boil the lemon in distilled water for 10 minutes in a glass pot with a cover. After it cools, drink one cup a day.

This is a powerful drink because the lemon's bioflavonoids and Vitamin C will go into the boiling liquid. When you drink this, you will get many bioflavonoids that you cannot get in any capsule or pill.

Psyllium

In previous chapters, I have discussed how to use psyllium. Psyllium is good to use as a temporary measure to get fiber in your diet immediately. Make sure you buy psyllium from a health-food store in the bulk area. Many of the commercial products have too many additives.

Take 2-3 teaspoon three times a day. You can put it in water or juice. Drink additional water, after drinking your glass of psyllium. Psyllium bulks up, and you want plenty of water to make it flow into the colon and not get stuck anywhere. Start with a small amount of psyllium, like a tablespoon. You will see how thick it gets in the water.

Sitting Pad

If you do a lot of sitting, then consider buying a thick soft pad or a doughnut-shaped pad to take the pressure off your anus area. You will definitely need this, if you have a medium or severe case of hemorrhoids.

Sitz Bath – Essential Oils

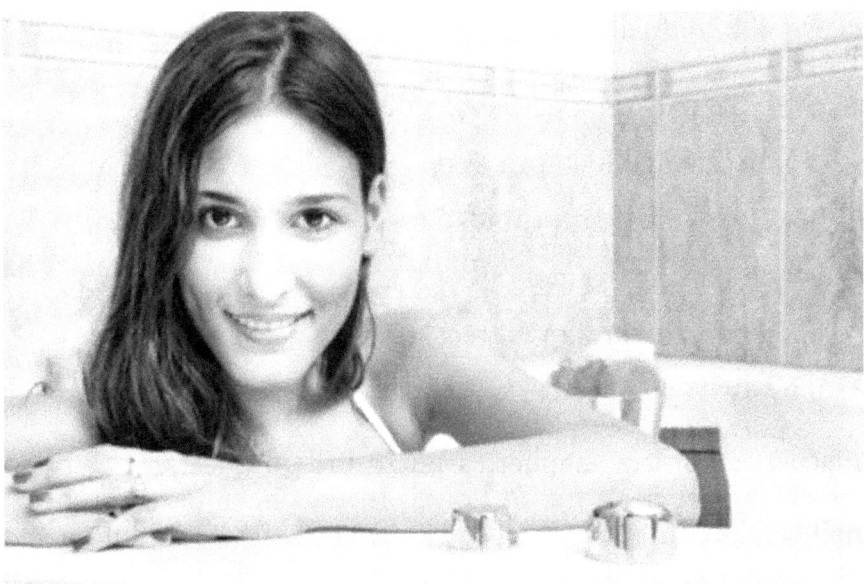

If you have swollen hemorrhoids, a sitz bath can help you reduce them and speed your recover. Fill a tub with warm or hot water. Use the temperature that will not irritate your hemorrhoids. Fill it so water reaches your hips or stomach, 6-8 inches. Then add 22 drops each of juniper and lavender essential oils.

Stir in the oils with your hand and then sit in the bath with your knee raised for 10-15 minutes three times a day. This position helps to bring more blood into your hemorrhoid area, which brings in more nutrients and to pulls out toxic waste.

After 15 minutes, take a shower with water as cold as you can take.

After this sitz bath, you can use one of the herbal ointments directly on your hemorrhoids and leave it on overnight.

Sitz Bath – Shepherd's Purse

The herb Shepherd's Purse can be used in sitz bath. This herb is useful in reducing,

- Internal and external bleeding
- Reducing blood pressure
- Relieving hemorrhoids
- Repairing wounds
- Reducing prolapsed rectum

Here's how to use it,

Place 1 oz. of the shepherd's purse in two quarts of distilled water and let it sit for 12 hours. In the morning or evening, boil this mixture and then strain it. Pour the liquid into a sitz tub or into a full bathtub. Stay in the tub for around 20 minutes and do this 2-3 times a day. You can also add juniper and lavender essential oils into the bath to make it more effective.

Witch Hazel and Basin

Prepare a small tub, container, or basin that you can sit in and add some warm distilled water. Add 1/4 cup of witch hazel liquid to the water. Sit in the small tub as long as you can and do it as often as you can. This will relieve your hemorrhoids in 3 to 4 days.

or, you can freeze witch hazel into small ice cubes, then wrap them with cheesecloth and press them against your hemorrhoids for 10- 15 minutes every hour. This will reduce the pain and swelling of your hemorrhoids.

Foot Reflexology

Foot reflexology is an overlook treatment, which is effective in removing energy blocks, which cause congestion such as hemorrhoids. Once energy blocks are removed blood and lymph liquid move freely, and congestion is unblocked. When congestion is relived, that part of the body will start to heal.

Foot reflexology can be very effective in relieving hemorrhoids, since they represent congestion of veins and tissue liquids. By applying constant or on and off pressure on the foot rectum reflex point, hemorrhoid healing can start to take place.

In her book, Hand Reflexology: Key to Perfect Health, 1976, Mildred Carter tells about her problem with hemorrhoids,
"I suffered from hemorrhoids for years and at times there was such excessive bleeding I thought I would bleed to death. Many times, I would get up and work all night because the pain was so severe I couldn't lie down or sit still. I used every kind of an ointment there was... I was introduced to reflexology by a friend ...when she touched the reflexes to the hemorrhoids on my heels, I nearly went through the ceiling from the pain... She showed me how to find these bottoms so I could massage them myself...in just two or three day I massage the soreness out and I have never had a recurrence of the disorder... I also have never stopped using reflexology."

The reflex point on your foot for hemorrhoids is along the bony edge of your heel as shown in the video just below.

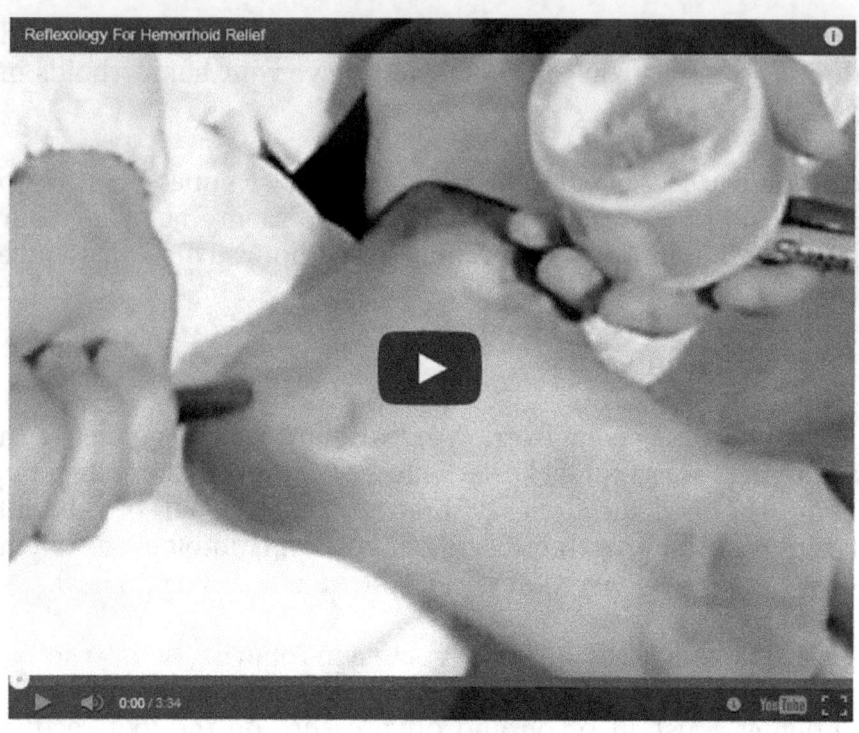

Or, go to
http://www.healingsamurai.net/page.asp?ID=65 to
watch the video.

If you have hemorrhoids, this area will have pain when you massage it. Massage this area slowly. Press down hard with your thumb or knuckles and hold for a bit, then inch over slightly to the next point and press again.

When you find a painful or sore area, work this area until it is no longer sore. This will take a few days, so keep at it.

Another way to work the hemorrhoid reflex points is to walk on your heels for 20 – 30 counts. If this is too painful just do it for, however, many steps you can do. Do this exercise morning and evening.

You can also do hand reflexology, using the following diagram.

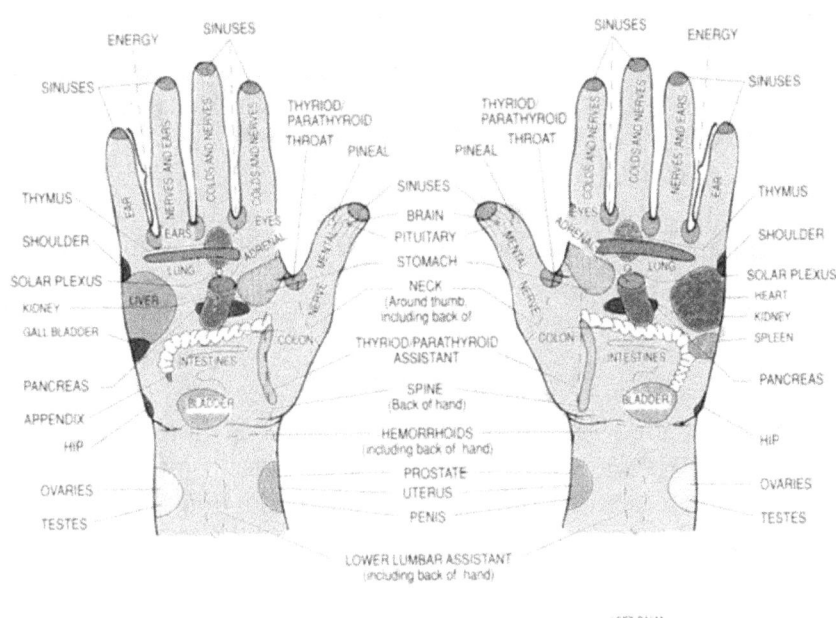

The hemorrhoid points are just below the hand and in the wrist area. Massage this are for 15 to 20 seconds in a circular motion, then go in a counter clock motion. Start slowly at first, then increase the pressure as is comfortable. To get the best results with reflexology look for a certified reflexologist to massage your feet and hands.

Sitting on the toilet

When go into the bathroom, go in there to have a bowel movement. Don't take a newspaper to read because that keeps you in there longer. Sitting on the toilet puts pressure on your rectum and anal veins and eventually leads to hemorrhoids or aggravates the hemorrhoids you already have. So, you don't want to sit there longer than necessary.

When sitting on the toilet, there are a few things you can do to help your stools come out easier. You don't want to strain or push hard. This will make your hemorrhoids worse.

Sit-up straight and lean back slightly

Raise your arms up above you, this helps to stretch and move your colon. Use a small stool to place your feet on to move your knees up a little. This takes off some of the pressure felt in your anal area. Move your stomach in and out to help stimulate your colon. Move side to side to stretch and move your colon. If you have a job where you have to sit all the time, get up and walk around every hour or as often as you can.

Exercise

Exercise is called for in helping to get rid of hemorrhoids. A good daily fast walk is the best. Yoga is very helpful, since it helps to stretch muscles, and revive circulation. Any exercise will be beneficial.

You can do all the things for preventing hemorrhoids and constipation, but if you do not exercise regularly, you are bound to get these aliments. So plan to exercise, it is good for life and not just good for hemorrhoids and constipation.

Visualization

If you have the ability to visualize and use affirmations to heal yourself, and many people do, you can use the following method.

In his book, Healthy Digestion the Natural Way, 2000, D. Lindsey Berkson outlines visualization,

- Lie down in a quiet place
- Become aware of your body
- Tighten your anus area a couple of times and breathe deeply
- Imagine a green ball of light the size of a baseball sitting on top of your head.
- With each breath you take, let the ball sink into your head to fill it up with the green light.

- Let the ball travel from the top of your head to the anal area.
- Feel the soothing and coolness as the green light fills your body and then your rectum area
- Focusing on your anus area, say as you inhale, HEAL and on exhaling say, REPAIR
- Repeat these words for a long as you like.

7: Heal Hemorrhoid With Vitamins and Nutrients

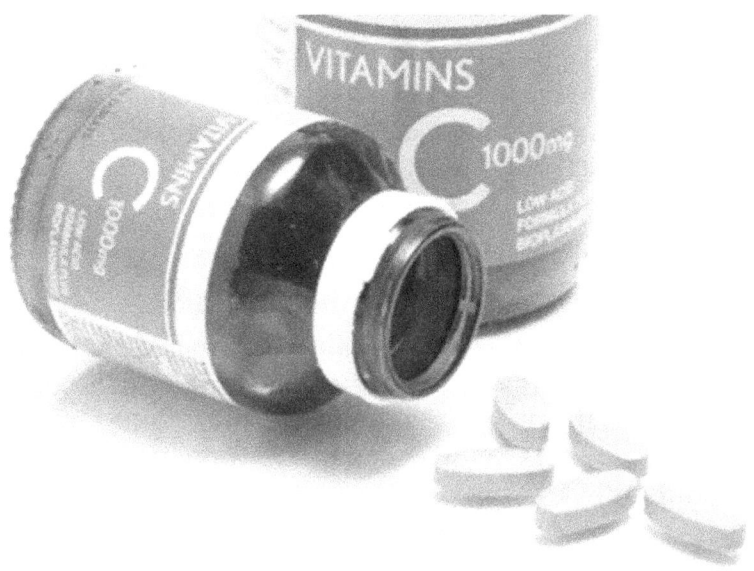

When you have hemorrhoids taking specific vitamins and nutrients is necessary for you to recover. Here is a list of nutrients to choose from. Pick four to five of them to add to your program. When you are sick, you need to double the amount of vitamins or nutrients you take. Just taking the normal amount is not good enough, when you are sick.

Always take vitamins during meal or after meal time. Taking them between meals can give you a stomach ache.

Vitamin A

Take a least 10,000 IU a day. Vitamin A is necessary for rebuilding tissue.

Vitamin C

Make sure you start taking vitamin C right away. Vitamin C

helps to build and strengthen blood vessel walls by maintaining the structure of collagen in the tissues and veins surrounding the rectum. It can also be used to soften your stools.

Take a minimum of 1000 mg vitamin C three times a day. Take more up to where you get diarrhea and them back off slightly on the dose. Some people start to get diarrhea with 1500mg and other can take up to 4000-5000mg or more without any problem.

Vitamin B Complex

Use a Vitamin B Complex – 50 or a –100, capsule three times a day. The B vitamins are good for digestion, which reduces stress and pressure on the rectum. But, make sure you take 100 mg of Vitamin B6 twice a day, and after you get relief, drop this amount to 75 mg per day.

Your urine will be deep yellow with the B vitamins. Your body will use the B vitamins it needs and excretes what it does not use in your urine.

Health tip: If you are pregnant, make sure you take this dose of Vitamin B6 since mostly likely you will be short on this Vitamin.

Vitamin E

Take a minimum of 400 IU of Vitamin E in the morning with your meal and 400 IU with your evening meal. Vitamin E improves your blood circulation and helps to rebuild and strengthen your artery walls.

Bioflavonoids

Health tip: Bioflavonoids have been found to be most effective in helping to relieve and eliminate the symptoms of hemorrhoids. They are useful in reducing enlarged veins in the rectum and in the legs (varicose veins.) Add them to your plan in eliminating hemorrhoids.

The bioflavonoids that have been used in clinical studies and have shown positive hemorrhoidal results are,

- Rutin – a bioflavonoid
- Daflon – a bioflavonoid that contain Diosmin and hesperidin, which are found in citrus fruits.
- Hydroxyethylrutosides (HER) or Oxerutins - a bioflavonoid that is a mixture of chemicals that comes from rutin –
- HER or Oxerutins may only be available from your doctor or a health care practitioner.

Rutin

Rutin is a bioflavonoid, which is effective in reducing hemorrhoids. It does this by strengthening and improving the permeability of the blood vessels and capillaries. Blood vessels that have a high efficiency of allowing nutrients and wastes to move in and out of their walls easily – permeability – allow the area involved to recover from illness quicker.

Here are some of the benefits of rutin:

- Provides nutritional support to the circulatory systems.
- Provides nutrition to the eye capillaries and is used for glaucoma
- Prevents recurrent bleeding caused by weakened blood vessels
- Prevents blood vessel walls becoming fragile

In addition to treatment for hemorrhoids, rutin has been found useful and effective for poor circulation, high blood pressure, varicose veins, capillary fragility, and other conditions where the blood vessels are weak.

In his booklet called Natural Remedies for what Ails You, 1985, Mark Bricklin shares some testimonials about the use of rutin,

"Last summer I was home visiting my mother. I had just returned from a long and very tiring trip, where I was on my feet all day every day. At this time, I was having terrible pains and chills, and bleeding from hemorrhoids. I had been having trouble for eight years, and the doctors were recommending surgery.

I had been in bed at my mother's house for three days when she started me on rutin tablets. In one week, my hemorrhoids were gone: no bleeding or swelling. It has been a year this month, and I have never been bothered again. –K.R., Oklahoma.' "

Foods that contain rutin are,

- Buckwheat
- Lemons
- Oranges
- Grapes
- Plums
- Apricots,
- Cherries,
- Blackberries,
- Green peppers,
- Currants
-

But, most foods do not contain enough rutin to help your hemorrhoids. So it is best to use a supplement.

There are, however, some herbs that are high in rutin, such as,
- Wild pansy flowers – one flower has up to 20 mg of

rutin

- Violets

- Eucalyptus leaf

- Mulberry leaf.

Here's where to get rutin,

Rutin Supplements or http://tinyurl.com/lztutkf

How to use rutin

Take from 30 to 80 mg of rutin three times a day. Use the high dose for severe cases and the lower dose for mild cases. Use Vitamin C with rutin to make rutin's curative powers even more effective.

You can experiment with the dose by taking up to 100 mg of rutin per day.

Magnesium

As mentioned before, lack of magnesium can cause constipation. The proper level of magnesium balanced with calcium is necessary for the colon and rectum to contract and relax as it does during peristaltic movement.

Since most processed foods contain little magnesium, it is usually necessary for you to take calcium and magnesium in a 2:1 or 1:1 ratio (A 500 mg of calcium to 250 mg magnesium capsule.)

Iron

If you have had excess bleeding from your hemorrhoids, then an iron supplement may be in order or at least add foods to your diet that contain iron.

Here some symptoms if you are low on iron:

- Fatigue – low energy
- Depression and irritability
- Fainting spells and headaches
- Itching
- Pale lips and skin
- Sore tongue, brittle nails
- Poor appetite
- Poor memory

Because iron helps to form hemoglobin, which delivers oxygen to your cells, the main symptoms you may have are tiredness depression, irritability and headaches. Oxygen is the element that burns the nutrients in your cells to give you energy.

Bleeding is one way of losing iron, but there are certain foods that block the absorption of iron. You should try to avoid these when you have bleeding hemorrhoids or other internal bleeding.

Here are the foods to avoid,

- Tea and coffee when taken with meals

- Ice cream, candy bars

- Sodas, beer

- Baked items

- The ETA additive

Calcium

If you are taking calcium with your meal, take them about an hour after your meal. In this way, you don't block the iron that is in your meal.

8: Foods That Relieve Hemorrhoids

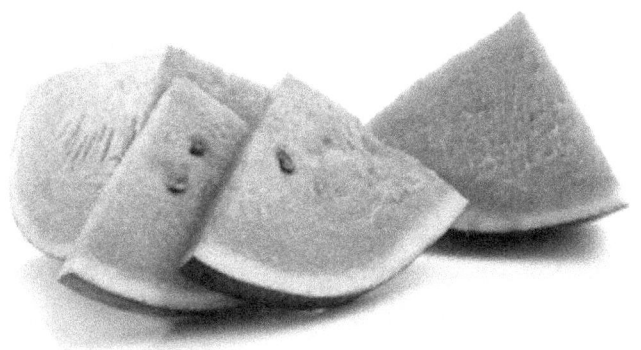

Foods to Avoid

Chili Peppers

It has been found that when you eat a lot of chili peppers that you can get a burning sensation in the rectum or anus. It is best to avoid eating too many peppers, especially if you have an advance case of hemorrhoids. Peppers are actually good for blood circulation and for healing ulcer. It is always the excess that creates problems in your body. So, don't avoid chili peppers if you like them.

Avoid the following foods:

- Coffee
- Alcohol
- Fats
- Animal products
- Red meat

Foods For Your hemorrhoids

A high-fiber diet obtained from raw fruits and vegetables, is what you need to preventing constipation and cure hemorrhoids.

If you have not been eating a lot of fiber, you need to add fiber slowly to your diet, especially if you add it by using bran. Increase your use of bran or oats over a couple of weeks.

If you add fiber to your diet with fruits and vegetables, you can add them freely without many problems. However, since your stomach will not be used to it, you may experience more gas for a week or two.

The following list of foods is good for helping cure or relieves hemorrhoids.

Juices

Juices are good for hemorrhoids, but especially dark berry juice mixed with equal parts of apple juice. The dark berry juices to use are,

Cherries, blackberries, blueberries

These berries contain "anthocyanins" and "proanthocyanidins" which reduce hemorrhoidal pain and swelling by toning and strengthening the hemorrhoidal veins. Drink at least one glass or more of this juice mixture each day.

Iron foods

Here are the foods that contain iron to help building up your blood or to keep iron in reserve, if you ever need it.

- Chicken liver, steamed crab
- Beef liver

- kelp
- Prunes
- Dried apricots
- Blackstrap molasses
- Spinach
- Sunflower seeds
- Pistachios
- Cashews, almonds, sesame seeds
- Baked potatoes
- Cooked Swiss chard
- Lima beans,
- Raisins
- Cooked broccoli
- Tuna

Cantaloupe

Cantaloupes and watermelon are one of the best foods you can eat. They have a good source of vitamins and minerals. They are high beta-carotene level and have anti-clogging properties. You can eat these two fruits together, but not with other fruits.

Ginger, Garlic, and Onion

Add these three herbs to your diet. Each one of these helps to break down fibrin. As I mentioned before fibrin creates inflammation and blood congestion by trying to repair arteries and veins.

Red and Black Currant Berries

Currants are high in Vitamin C, rutin, and minerals. This makes their juice valuable in clearing hemorrhoids. They also have a small amount of the fatty acid GLA, which produces prostaglandin that control body pain.

This juice is also excellent for cleansing the liver and blood. Good liver function is necessary for maintaining a healthy

colon, rectum and anus.

Drink 2-3 glasses a day of red or black currant berries.

Pomegranate Juice

Although pomegranate juice may be hard to find, it is quite useful in reducing hemorrhoids, because of its strong astringency. Saturate a cotton ball with pomegranate juice and push it slightly into your rectum.

If you have pinworms, the tannins in pomegranate juice will help you get rid of them. You can also drink the juice. During the summer, I have on occasion found pomegranate juice at a farmer's market. It is slightly tart, but it is easy to drink. But, it's hard to drink more than a glass full without starting a stomach upset.

Oranges and bananas

Eat 2-3 oranges and 2 bananas a day. Oranges provide vitamin C, bioflavonoids, and fiber. Bananas provide minerals that help to strengthen tissue and have plenty of fiber.
Bananas can also be steamed to give more relief and even eliminate hemorrhoids.

Steam two not quite ripe bananas with their peel until they are soft. Eat two in the morning and two in the evening.

Oils

At every meal, use olive oil, flax seed oil, and apple cider vinegar in your salad. In your soups, use olive and flax seed oil or other food dishes where they are appropriate. Or, at the end of each meal, take your capsule of fish oil.

Fish oil is probably one of the most important oils to use daily. Go to my newsletter to read the article I wrote about this Fish

Oil.

Natural Remedies Thatwork Newsletter Website

Papaya

Papaya is an excellent fruit to eat. It has good mineral content, fiber, and has enzymes to digest protein.

Here some foods to eat

Use the following foods to help reduce hemorrhoidal bleeding:

Alfalfa
Dark-green leafy vegetables
Blackstrap molasses

Flax seeds – are high in omega-3 oils, which reduce inflammation and pain. They are also high in fiber. Lima and butter beans are high in iron, which help to build more blood. If you have bleeding hemorrhoids, adding lima beans to your diet would be a good choice.

Sweet potatoes provide fiber, B vitamins, iron, potassium and many other vitamins and minerals. This is a good body building food.

Health Alert: If after trying different hemorrhoidal remedies listed here for up to two weeks and your hemorrhoids not have shrunk or gone away, you might consider seeing a doctor. You need to find out if your hemorrhoids exist because of a more serious medical condition.

See your doctor right away if you have a lot of anal bleeding, a lot of blood in your stools, heavy pain, or fecal incontinence.

Salads

Eat plenty of salads with raw vegetable. Both vegetables and fruits that are heated where the natural enzymes are destroyed also turn calcium into an inorganic form. In the body, this inorganic form is not useable.

These excess inorganic calcium moves into body areas that are sluggish and deposits causing inflammation and disease. One area it migrates to is the rectum, where it activates the formation of hemorrhoids.

So eat plenty of raw vegetables sprinkled with apple cider vinegar. There you have it. Plenty of remedies that can give you temporary relief, reduce bleeding, reduce swelling, eliminate itching, and cure your hemorrhoids.

9: Liver Cleansing That Reduces Hemorrhoids

Liver Cleanse

If you have reoccurring hemorrhoids, you may have a congested or weak liver. It is recommended that you use a liver-cleansing product.

Even if you do not have reoccurring hemorrhoids, you will benefit greatly by doing a 5 or 7-day liver cleanse.

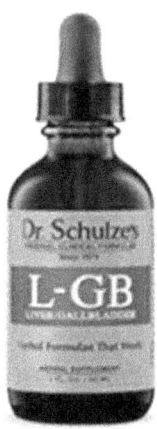

Using **Dr. Schulze's Liver cleanse** is the best way to do your liver cleanse.

But, an alternative way to do a liver cleanse is to use This **7-Day Liver Cleanse** or go to **http://www.renewlife.com/7-day-liver-cleanse**.

About Your Liver

Your liver is central to how your body functions. If your liver is sluggish, clogged, or diseased, you will be open to many different diseases, such are constipation, high cholesterol, IBS, high blood sugar, asthma, skin rashes, acne, allergies and more.

Your liver is a detoxifying organ. Because of the tremendous pollution that is in the environment and in everything you eat and drink, your liver is usually overloaded. Your liver is called upon to eliminate all of this pollution and at some point becomes unable to do this. When this happens, your liver allows various pollutants to enter your blood. This is when other organs become compromised, and cells and body liquids become contaminated. Over time, you become diseased.

Liver distress

So what causes your liver to become distressed? Your liver becomes distress, when you eat processed foods, food in packages, sugar, artificial sweeteners, caffeine, dips, breads, cookies, and hydrogenated oil. It becomes distressed when you don't have a healthy diet.

A Liver Diet

Your liver likes fresh, whole fruits and vegetables or cooked lightly. It likes cooked grains and legumes, raw nuts, and seeds.

It likes food with fiber. You need around 35 grams of fiber every day. In your colon, fiber absorbs excess cholesterol and estrogen and prevents it from being reabsorbed into your blood. When reabsorbed estrogen gets into your blood, it becomes active and disturbs the balance of your hormones.
Fiber is also necessary to prevent constipation. Fiber absorbs water in your colon and prevents your stools from becoming hard and difficult to move through your colon.

Enzymes that digest your food come from fresh produce and from within your body. If you eat mostly processed foods, you will be using up your enzymes. When you are low on body enzymes, you will decrease your ability to digest foods. This will cause poor digestion, which creates acid wastes that your liver has to deal with.

Detoxifying Your Liver

Your liver needs plenty of fruits and vegetables every day, to detoxify. This produce has the fiber, nutrients, and antioxidants that your liver uses, to cleanse itself and other body organs.

Your liver also needs to see a reduction in the consumption of bad fatty acids, such as hydrogenated and partial hydrogenated oil found in all junk food. Hydrogenated oils are deadly and lead to cardiovascular diseases.

10: A Hemorrhoid Program to Get You Started

The first thing you need to do is get your bowel movements back to normal. When you have a bowel movement, you don't want to strain or push. The following steps will help you get you started on eliminating constipation.

Start through each step and start doing a little on each step each week. Each week do a little more and so on. After a month or two, you should be on your way to living and eating in a different manner.

Hemorrhoid Program

Constipation Step by Step

In this program, you will start with eliminating constipation or having easier bowel movements. As you deal with constipation, you can at the same time deal with the hemorrhoids.

Here are the steps.

1. Start drinking more distilled water. This can be in the form of eating more fruits, herbal teas, fruit or vegetable juices or just plain water.

2. Eat more natural fiber. You will get more fiber as you eat fruits. But, you also need to eat a salad with your lunch and dinner. Eat raw vegetable salads. Try to get the different color vegetables in your salad. Eat oats, bran, and other whole-grain products on occasion only.

3. Eat less protein and eliminating white bread and milk

from you diet. If you insist on eating bread make sure it's with vegetables, so that as the bread goes through your colon, you will have fiber with it

4. Start reducing the processed foods that you eat. This is a gradual step. You don't and you probably can't stop eating this type of food instantly. Every week stop eating a specific processed food.

5. Choose a natural constipation remedy like MSM, Aloe Vera drink or capsules, cayenne capsules or Oxypowder. Oxypowder is a powerful colon cleanser that helps you remove fecal matter that is collecting in your colon and doesn't want to come out. Within a couple of weeks your colon will be clean and ready for you to start new without constipation.

6. Take a mineral and vitamin complex to strengthen your colon.

7. Always use digestive enzymes and probiotics. The enzymes help you digest your food better, and you will live longer and the same goes for probiotics or good bacteria. Your body needs good bacteria to keep you healthy and free of colon problems. You always have bacteria in your intestinal tract, but you want to have more good bacteria than bad, otherwise you will always be sick.

8. Use good oils in your salad or soups. Take olive oil and flax seed oil and mix it into your salad. You can also add it to your soups, after it has cooled down a little. Be creative on where you use these oils. Or, you can supplement with fish oil, so you can get plenty of omega-3 oil.

9. Get exercise every day. Just start slowly, if you are not exercising. You can walk briskly around the block to start, but just start and then do it every day at the same time.

10. If you are an anxious person and have a lot of stress, you need to do something about this. Stress is really the number-one killer disease. Most disease comes from stress, but this is not listed as number one, since doctors don't study the cause of the many deadly diseases.

Hemorrhoid Step by Step

1. Get some aloe vera gel, fresh or in a bottle. Make sure it's whole leaf aloe vera. This type uses all the plant and is more potent. Apply this to your rectum. Apply this as often as you can. If you are home do it every hour.

   You can also take aloe vera capsules. This will help your digestion and constipation. If you like the aloe vera fruit juice, you can drink this.

2. Start taking capsules to strengthen your vein walls in your rectum. As an alternate, you can use the Collinsonia capsules. They have an excellent history with hemorrhoids. Add to this a good dose of vitamin C, at least 4000 to 5000 mg.

3. Get some comfrey root powder and horse chestnut powder and mix them with olive oil, almond oil, or coconut oil. Create a paste then apply it to your rectum. Use a pad to keep the paste in place.

   Now, you can buy the comfrey root ointment, and you can try that. Experiment with different things, until you find what works for you.

4. If the Comfrey root product does not work for you try the Veri-Gone Salve.

5. Using the Zinc ointment is a must, so use this in combination with the other ointments or salves. You can just mix in a bit of zinc ointment with the comfrey root or other ointments. There are other ointments you can use, but this will get you started.

6. Get some liquid chlorophyll and have a morning drink with lemon juice. This will help you get rid of toxins and cleanse your body every day. This also good for cleansing your liver.

7. Using digestive enzymes every day is a must. Do this with probiotics. These nutrients will help you completely digest your food, so that you don't easily get constipation.

8. If you are familiar with reflexology and enjoy this, then now is the time to use this with your hemorrhoid condition.

9. Take these vitamins with your other capsules during or after your meals, vitamin A, C, B, and E. You should be taking these anyway all the time.

10. Consider taking rutin, it has been shown to be effective with hemorrhoids.

11. Look over the chapter on "Foods Relieve Hemorrhoids." Add these foods to your diet.

12. If you have been on a junk food diet for a long time, then you need to do a liver cleanse. Get a five-day kit to cleanse your liver. If you have been eating healthy off

and on, then you might not need to do a liver cleanse. However, it's always best to do this cleanse, since it will improve your health.

Finally,

You have many different herbal treatments to choose from. Look over the hemorrhoid gels, ointments, herbs, or supplements. Try the ones that you think will help you and use them for a week. If you see no improvement, then try another combination. Some creams, ointments, or gels are more effective than others and this depends on what your condition is.

Use both an external and internal treatment at the same time. You want to work from the outside and inside.

You also want to make a change in the things and the way you eat. Start eating more fruits and vegetables and fewer meat products.

Remember, that the way you have been living your life to this point has created your hemorrhoid, so you need to change what you are doing, if you want to eliminate and not have another bout with them.

Start trying to eat more fruits and juices and oats in the morning. Get away from eating a heavy breakfast, such as eggs, potatoes, ham, bread, butter, and jelly. A fruit breakfast helps to detoxify you and will you get regular.

There you have it plenty of information for getting rid of your hemorrhoids and constipation. I don't expect you to make all these changes at once. Make changes weekly. Of course, if you have chronic constipation, then use some natural remedies to help to clear out your colon, such as **Oxypowder** or go here **http://tinyurl.com/kqalcsd** .

11: About The Author And Other Resources

Get one of my best kindle books *free* below:

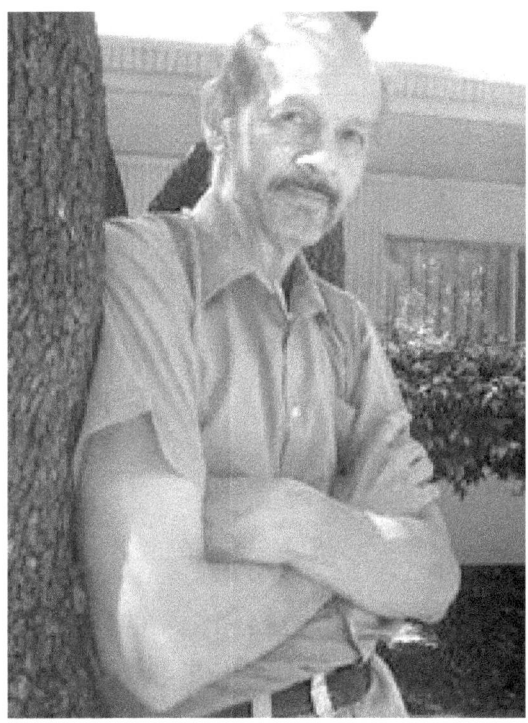

http://www.natural-remedies-thatwork.com

Rudy Silva is a natural consultant nutritionist educated in the United States in Nutrition and Physics. He is a graduate from the San Jose State University in California. He is author of 45 other books on natural remedies. He has authored a newsletter in natural remedies for over 4 years.

Resource page
Here are some of the other kindle e-books about natural

remedies that have been written by this author. You can see the entire list at:

http://tinyurl.com/b2f7wd3

Acne Remedies
Best natural acne treatments: Acne facial

Constipation Remedies
How To Relieve Constipation With Fruits

Essential Fatty Acids
Amazing Fish Oil Benefits Revealed

Nutrition Remedies
Fantastic Alkaline Fruit Benefits Revealed

Magnesium Nutrition Revealed

Best Nutrition Health Practices

Potassium Health Secrets Revealed

Phosphorus, The Best Brain Food

A Sodium Diet (What You Must Know About Sodium)

Stomach Remedies
Acid Reflux: Fast and Easy Cures For Acid Reflux

How To Do Natural Colon Cleansing

Misc. Remedies

Iron Deficiency Anemia

What Is A Hiatus Hernia

Best Varicose Vein Treatments?

Men's Health

Best Impotence Health Diet

Weight loss
Ten (10) Day Quick Success Weight Loss Program

To see all of the kindle books written by this author, go to this the Authors Profile Page or this URL:

http://tinyurl.com/b2f7wd3

If you need support or want to promote any of his e-books, please contact him at rss41@yahoo.com and expect a reply within 24 hours. He looks forward to hearing from you.

Give A Review

And, don't for get to give a review for this e-book at Amazon so that others can gain the benefits of what is in this e-book.

To you, for losing weight, creating better health and more happiness in your life,

Rudy S Silva

www.ingramcontent.com/pod-product-compliance
Lightning Source LLC
Chambersburg PA
CBHW070606290526
45790CB00002B/802